YOUR KNOWLEDGE HAS VALUE

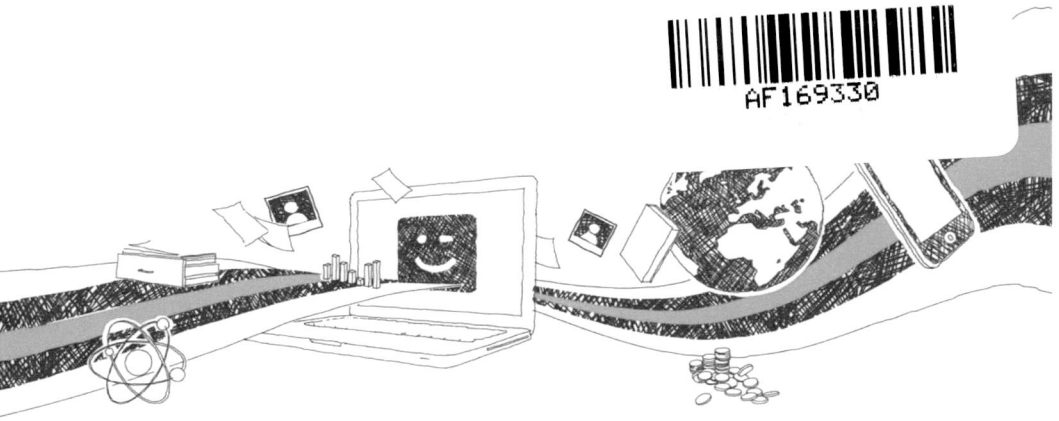

- We will publish your bachelor's and
  master's thesis, essays and papers

- Your own eBook and book -
  sold worldwide in all relevant shops

- Earn money with each sale

Upload your text at www.GRIN.com
and publish for free

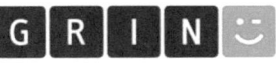

Bibliographic information published by the German National Library:

The German National Library lists this publication in the National Bibliography; detailed bibliographic data are available on the Internet at http://dnb.dnb.de .

This book is copyright material and must not be copied, reproduced, transferred, distributed, leased, licensed or publicly performed or used in any way except as specifically permitted in writing by the publishers, as allowed under the terms and conditions under which it was purchased or as strictly permitted by applicable copyright law. Any unauthorized distribution or use of this text may be a direct infringement of the author s and publisher s rights and those responsible may be liable in law accordingly.

Imprint:

Copyright © 2018 GRIN Verlag
Print and binding: Books on Demand GmbH, Norderstedt Germany
ISBN: 9783668636132

This book at GRIN:

https://www.grin.com/document/388411

Patrick Kimuyu

Parkinson's Disease and Its Management

GRIN Verlag

GRIN - Your knowledge has value

Since its foundation in 1998, GRIN has specialized in publishing academic texts by students, college teachers and other academics as e-book and printed book. The website www.grin.com is an ideal platform for presenting term papers, final papers, scientific essays, dissertations and specialist books.

Visit us on the internet:

http://www.grin.com/

http://www.facebook.com/grincom

http://www.twitter.com/grin_com

Parkinson's Disease and Its Management

Name: Patrick Kimuyu

Introduction 2
Epidemiology 2
Pathophysiology 3
Signs and Symptoms 4
Diagnosis 4
Treatment 5
Conclusion 7
References 8

Introduction

Parkinson's disease (PD) is considered as a progressive disorder of the central nervous system, and it is characterized by difficulties in movement. This disorder is also referred to as the shaking palsy owing to the tremors experienced by the patients (Lyons & Pahwa 2007). It is one of the most challenging motor system disorders because it is both chronic and progressive; implying that symptoms emerge and worsen over time. Therefore, the management of Parkinson's disease presents an immense challenge to healthcare professionals, as well as families and relatives of patients suffering from the disease. Currently, there is no cure for Parkinson's disease; thus, treatment approaches focus on reducing the severity of its symptoms.

Aetiology of Parkinson's disease remains uncertain (Lippincott Williams & Wilkins 2005). However, environmental and genetic factors have been hypothesized as the principal cause of the disease condition. It is believed that a combination of environmental and genetic factors account for the onset of Parkinson's disease in most people. Some of the most significant environmental risk factors associated with Parkinson's disease include exposure to pesticides and herbicides, proximity to industries, and consumption of well water (Wirdefeldt, Adami, Cole, Trichopoulos & Mandel 2011). On the other hand, evidence indicates that genetic factors account for 10% of Parkinson's disease cases (Hauser 2014). Berkris, Mata and Zabetian (2010, p. 228) report "Mutations in 6 genes (SNCA, LRRK2, PRKN, DJ1, PINK1, and ATP13A2) have conclusively been shown to cause familial parkinsonism; common variation in 3 genes (MAPT, LRRK2, and SNCA) and loss-of-function mutations in GBA have been well-validated as susceptibility factors for PD." This report provides an overview of Parkinson's disease and its management.

Epidemiology

Epidemiological studies indicate that Parkinson's disease affects about 1% of people order than 60 years. It is estimated that the prevalence of Parkinson's disease is 120 cases per 100,000 people, and its incidence rate ranges from 4.5 to 21 cases in the same population. However, the prevalence of the disease exhibits demographic trends. For instance, its prevalence rate in men is 1.5 times more than in women. On the other hand, this disease exhibits racial and ethnic trends in which the Europeans and Americans are more affected than Asian communities (Tan & Louis 2013). Hispanics are known to have the highest prevalence rate of the disease (Muangpaisan, Hori & Brayne 2009). Currently, one million Americans, 9,000 Chinese and 127,000 people in UK are suffering from Parkinson's disease.

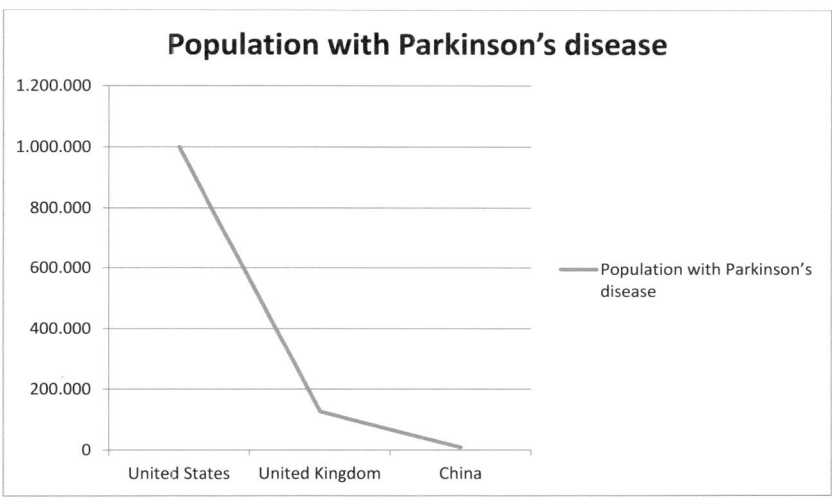

Pathophysiology

From a pathological perspective, it is relatively difficult to explain the pathophysiology of Parkinson's disease because its neuropathologic trends have not been understood. However, there are some parameters that suggest the progression of the disease condition. Some of these parameters include the presence of Lewy neurites and Lewy bodies, as well as, the absence of some dopaminergic neurons in the brain. Evidence indicates that the pigmented dopaminergic neurons which are predominantly found in the substantia nigra of the ventral lateral region of the brain disappear before the onset of Parkinson's disease symptoms. This situation has been identified to occur in 60% to 80% of Parkinson's disease cases (Hauser 2014).

On the other hand, Lewy bodies have been found to play a pathological role in the progression of Parkinson's disease. This is so because the prevalence of incidental Lewy bodies and neurites increase with age. As such, they are believed to have pathological influence during the pre-symptomatic phase of the disease.

Signs and Symptoms

In practice, the symptoms observed in Parkinson's disease patients are attributable to the changes in the motor circuit. Ordinarily, normal movement is coordinated by the cortical output which is usually modulated by the basal ganglia motor circuit. In Parkinson's disease, motor circuit from the cerebral cortex is impaired owing to the absence of dopaminergic neurons in the feedback pathway. It is believed that the inhibitory output that occurs in the thalamocortical pathway is responsible for the suppression of the movement observed in Parkinson's patients. This occurs because dopamine is the principal neurotransmitter involved in the direct and indirect pathways of the basal ganglia-thalamocortical motor circuit. Therefore, the decrease in dopamine levels in Parkinson's disease has been found to be responsible for the pathophysiological mechanisms which lead to the emergence of the main symptoms (Hauser 2014).

Parkinson's disease is manifested through an array of signs and symptoms. However, this disease is characterized by four principal signs: tremor of the limbs and jaws, slowness of movement (bradykinesia), stiffness of the trunk and the limbs (rigidity), and impaired coordination and balance (postural instability) (Lippincott Williams & Wilkins 2005). These signs and symptoms are experienced at various stages of the disease progression. Some of the symptoms experienced at the initial stages of Parkinson's disease include decreased facial expression, decreased arm swing, tremor, and a subtle decrease in dexterity. In addition, sleep disturbances, slowness in thinking, malaise, and rapid eye movements are considered as some of the most significant symptoms of Parkinson's disease (Simuni & Sethi 2008). Autonomic dysfunctions such as constipation, sexual dysfunction, sweating abnormalities, and seborrheic dermatitis are experienced at the initial stages of the disease. Ordinarily, these symptoms are manifested before the onset of motor signs. Some of the most significant motor signs include typical asymmetry, resting tremor especially in an upper extremity, progressively flexed axial posture, and balance impairment which occur at advanced stages of Parkinson's disease.

Diagnosis

Diagnosis of Parkinson's disease is associated with immense difficulties because there are no laboratory biomarkers which have been developed for the diagnosis of the condition (Hauser 2014). However, radiologic, histological and CSF testing provide significant approaches to the diagnosis of the condition. Olfactory testing is also considered as one of the most reliable diagnostic approaches for Parkinson's disease (Tolosa, Gaig, Santamaría & Compta 2009).

Radiological studies include Magnetic Resonance Imaging (MRI), Positron Emission Topography (PET) and Single-Photon Emission Computed Tomography (SPECT). MRI is usually used for differential diagnosis of Parkinson's disease in which tumours, strokes, hydrocephalus, lesions of Wilson disease and multi-infarct state are excluded. It is also useful in placing a thalamic stimulator. On the other hand, PET and SPECT scanning are useful in identifying abnormalities in the brain. These diagnostic approaches employ the measurement of dopamine levels in the brain. Therefore, high dopamine levels indicate the decrease of dopaminergic neurons which is a characteristic of Parkinson's disease.

Another significant approach to the diagnosis of Parkinson's disease is the use of histological tests. Histologic slides are investigated for the presence of Lewy bodies through Alpha-synuclein staining. Ideally, the presence of pigmented Lewy bodies in histologic slides confirms the diagnosis of Parkinson's disease. In theory, Parkinson's disease is believed to be a synucleinopathy; thus, Alpha-synuclein appears polymerized. Lumbar puncture is also used for the diagnosis of Parkinson's disease. This involves the removal of cerebrospinal fluid from the patients for culture and microscopic examination. In practice, the removal of 20 mL of CSF is usually followed by a significant improvement of the clinical signs (Hauser 2014).

In Parkinson's disease, homeopathy plays a significant role in addressing the disease consequences on patients. One of its benefits to patients is the restoration of gut flora balance. This approach ensures that the patient's body does not experience changes in homeostasis processes; thus, enabling them to cope with the disease symptoms. However, there are some complications which are common during homeopathic treatment that requires immediate attention of a general practitioner. Some of these complications include difficulty in swallowing, hallucinations, and the occurrence of cognitive dysfunction.

Treatment

Currently, there are different treatment option for Parkinson's disease including medication, surgery, physiotherapy and occupational therapy. However, medication and surgery have been the main orthodox medical treatment approaches in the management of the disease. The pharmacologic treatment of this disease is usually divided into two main therapies: symptomatic and neuroprotective therapy. Symptomatic therapy is intended to address the symptoms associated with Parkinson disease, whereas neuroprotective therapy focuses on slowing, blocking or reversing disease progression. Some of the most common therapeutic agents used for the symptomatic therapy include Levodopa, dopamine agonists and anticholinergic agents. On the other hand, neuroprotective therapy involves Selegiline, Rasagiline and Monoamine Oxidase-B inhibitors (Samii, Nutt & Ransom 2004).

Surgery is the second common treatment option for Parkinson's disease. Currently, Deep brain stimulation seems to have gained popularity owing to its reliability. It is apparent that this procedure does not cause destruction to the brain tissue, and it can be adjusted accordingly as the disease progresses. In addition, this procedure allows the application of bilateral procedures without adverse implications, besides being reversible unlike other surgery procedures which are not reversible. It is reported that DBS is useful in patients with unstable medication responses, especially in advanced Parkinson's disease. It also reduces tremor, rigidity and involuntary movements.

On the other hand, lesion surgeries such as thalamotomy, pallidotomy and subthalamotomy serve as reliable treatment options for Parkinson's disease. These surgeries involve the destruction of target regions of the thalamus to alleviate the signs of Parkinson's disease. For instance, the destruction of the ventralis intermedius through thalamotomy relieves tremor, whereas bradykinesia and rigidity are relieved through pallidotomy in which globus pallidus interna is destroyed. Therefore, surgery is usually favoured over pharmacologic treatment in situations where the patient is not responsive to medication (Knott 2013).

In the treatment of Parkinson's disease, Levodopa, dopamine agonists and Monoamine oxidase-B inhibitors are used as the main therapeutic remedies. In practice, Levodopa is the mainstay of treatment for Parkinson's patients from the onset of the disease symptoms to advanced stages. This agent is usually absorbed by neurons in the brain where it is converted into dopamine; thus, improving signal transmission. As a result, Levodopa helps in improving movement in Parkinson's patients. In most cases, Levodopa is administered in combination with additional medications such as Carbidopa or Benserazide (Stocchi, Rascol, Kieburtz et al. 2010). The role of the additional medications is to prevent Levodopa's breakdown during its transportation to the brain through the blood stream. In addition, these medications help in reducing the side effects of Levodopa including vomiting, dizziness, nausea, and tiredness. Despite the potency of Levodopa in the treatment of Parkinson's disease which leads to dramatic improvements, its effects are not long-lasting. As such, Levodopa dosage is supposed to be increased over the time, especially after the first year of therapeutic therapy. This dosage increase has adverse consequences to Parkinson's patients. Some of these consequences are jerky muscle movements, commonly referred to as dyskinesia and 'on-off' effects.

Dopamine agonists have similar effects to those of Levodopa because they are substitutes for dopamine in the brain. In practice, dopamine agonists are effective in treating early Parkinson's disease symptoms. The rationale for their use during early Parkinson is that they do not cause involuntary movements as it is the case with Levodopa. Therefore, dopamine agonists can be used for the treatment of early Parkinson's disease as alternatives for Levodopa. It is also logical to use Levodopa in combination with dopamine agonists, in order to lower the dosage of Levodopa; thus, preventing the development of its adverse side effects. Another commonly used therapeutic remedy for Parkinson's disease is Monoamine oxidase-B inhibitors. For instance, Selegiline prevents the oxidation of dopamine by inhibiting the activity of Monoamine oxidase-B enzyme. As a result, adequate dopamine levels are maintained; thus, reducing problems in movement. Selegiline is believed to improve the symptoms, more or less the same as Levodopa or dopamine agonists (Caslake, Macleod, Ives, Stowe & Counsell 2009).

From a professional perspective, patients should take diets with an adequate amount of salt to prevent cases of low blood pressure (NHS 2014).

Conclusion

Parkinson's disease is considered as one of the public health issues affecting the population. An adjunctive advice to people suffering from Parkinson's disease should address physical, speech and dietary problems. Patients should engage in movement and exercise, in order to relieve joint pain and muscle stiffness. This improves their fitness levels; thus, enabling them to manage their day-to-day activities. Secondly, diet plays a significant role in the management of all diseases, and dietary changes for patients with Parkinson's disease are recommended. For instance, the consumption of diets rich in fiber accompanied by enough fluids reduces constipation.

References

Berkris, L, Mata, I & Zabetian, C 2010, The Genetics of Parkinson Disease, *Journal of Geriatric Psychiatry and Neurology*, vol. 23, no. 4, pp. 228-242.

Caslake, R, Macleod, A, Ives, N, Stowe, R & Counsell, C 2009, Monoamine oxidase B inhibitors versus other dopaminergic agents in early Parkinson's disease, *Cochrane Database Syst Rev.* vol. 4, p. CD006661.

Hauser, R 2014, *Parkinson Disease*, viewed 23 July 2014, <http://emedicine.medscape.com/article/1831191-overview#showall>

Knott, L 2013, *Parkinson's Disease Management*, viewed 23 July 2014, <http://www.patient.co.uk/doctor/parkinsons-disease-management>

Lippincott Williams & Wilkins 2005, *Pathophysiology: A 2-in-1 Reference for Nurses*, New York, NY: Lippincott Williams & Wilkins.

Lyons, K & Pahwa, R 2007, *Handbook of Parkinson's disease*, Fourth Edition, Boca Raton, Fl: CRC Press.

Muangpaisan, W, Hori, H & Brayne, C 2009, Systemic review of the prevalence and incidence of Parkinson's disease in Asia, *J Epidermiol*, vol. 19, no. 5, pp. 281-93.

NHS 2014, *Parkinson's disease – Treatment*, viewed 23 July 2014, <http://www.nhs.uk/Conditions/Parkinsons-disease/Pages/treatment.aspx>

Samii, A, Nutt, JG & Ransom, BR 2004, Parkinson's disease. *Lancet*, vol. 363, no. 9423, pp. 1783–1793.

Simuni, T & Sethi, K 2008, Nonmotor manifestations of Parkinson's disease, *Ann Neurol*, vol. 64 no. 2, pp. S65-80.

Stocchi, F, Rascol, O, Kieburtz, K et al 2010, Initiating levodopa/carbidopa therapy with and without entacapone in early Parkinson disease: the STRIDE-PD study, *Ann Neurol.*, vol. 68, no. 1, pp. 18-27.

Tan, F & Louis, C 2013, Epidemiology of Parkinson's disease, *Neurology Asia*, vol. 18, no. 3, pp. 231 – 238, viewed 23 July 2014, <http://www.neurology-asia.org/articles/neuroasia-2013-18(3)-231.pdf>

Tolosa, E, Gaig, C, Santamaría, J & Compta, Y 2009, Diagnosis and the premotor phase of Parkinson disease, *Neurology*, vol. 72, no. 7, pp. S12-20.

Wirdefeldt, K, Adami, HO, Cole, P, Trichopoulos, D & Mandel, J 2011, Epidemiology and aetiology of Parkinson's disease: a review of the evidence. *Eur J Epidemiol*, vol. 26, no. 1, pp: S1-58.

YOUR KNOWLEDGE HAS VALUE

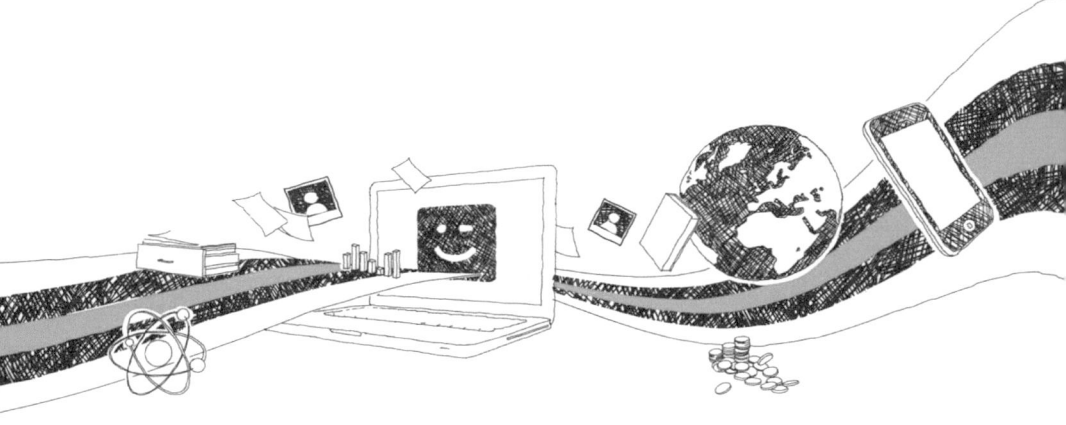

- We will publish your bachelor's and master's thesis, essays and papers

- Your own eBook and book - sold worldwide in all relevant shops

- Earn money with each sale

Upload your text at www.GRIN.com
and publish for free

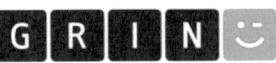